Natural Home Remedies for Shingles

By: Alyson Rodgers

Published by:
Alyson Rodgers and Random Technologies
4409 HOFFNER AVENUE, 347
Belle Isle, FL 32812

Disclaimer

Table of Contents

Introduction

So you're dealing with Shingles. Whether you're here for yourself or a loved one, you've come to the right place. No need to be embarrassed, this guide is going to walk you through the practical ways which you can use to get rid of your Shingles – quickly and effectively.

The tips in the guide are primarily natural, and lifestyle related. Be aware, this does not mean they're easy! Some are and some are not, the point is that these tips are available to cure Shingles.

Disclaimer
ALWAYS seek out a doctor's advice before proceeding with advice taking on the treatment of Shingles, this guide is no exception.

This guide is provided for educational and informational purposes, and should not substitute professional medical care. By agreeing to proceed, you are releasing myself and my company from any and all responsibility surrounding health effects of the individuals applying these teachings.

What is Shingles?

Before you take on the job of treating a disease, I think it's worth taking the time to do a bit of research and understand it. If you're thinking the same thing, you're in the right place. This guide will be all about understanding so that you can treat.

The Herpes Zoster Virus

So what exactly is Shingles? Simply put, Shingles is the Herpes Zoster virus. This virus moves throughout the body, beginning in the nose and lymph nodes, and travelling to other major organs like the liver and the spleen, tapping on your sensory tissue all the way along. It will continue to spread until stopped, by medication or by treatments like the ones outlined in this guide, and can ultimately reach the bloodstream and even your spinal cord.

Nasty bit of business, huh? In terms of what it looks like, Shingles has become known as the second bout of Chicken Pox. Chicken pox often affects younger people, as it is highly contagious but you can only get it once. Shingles will stay with you until you treat it by contrast.

The thing that confuses a lot of people is that the virus can switch between active and inactive states, and just because it's inactive does not mean you do not have it. Be aware that when visible, it is active, and at its most contagious – but having it crust over and disappear does not mean that your Shingles is gone.

Who it Affects

It primarily affects the elderly and those aging (adults). This could well be linked to the cause of Shingles, a weakened immune system.

The immune system is weakened by disease, unhealthy lifestyle, stress, damage from medications, and age. Indeed, age is a significant risk factor for developing Shingles.

> NOTE: You can still get Shingles even if you're vaccinated, the vaccination merely serves to weaken the disease.

How it Moves

In terms of how it passes, Shingles has been classified as being very contagious, particularly through coughs and sneezes of those suffering from the disease.

Symptoms of Shingles

Common Symptoms of Shingles
- Abdominal pain
- Aches (particularly in the muscles)
- Chills
- Coughing
- Delirium
- Diarrhea
- Difficulty breathing
- Eye irritation
- Fatigue that persists
- Fever
- Headaches
- Irritability
- Infection
- Loss of appetite
- Nausea
- Painful rash
- Phototobia (sensitivity to light)
- Red spots along the skin, indicating potential presence of rash
- Sensitive skin, indicating potential oncoming of rash
- Tenderness in the lymph nodes
- Throat irritation
- Tingling under the skin

- Urination issues
- Weight loss/weight gain

There are many symptoms of Shingles, the rash is just the most famously easy to diagnose. The truth is that if you're already fevered and seeing red spots on your skin, you can get checked out before the painful rash kicks in and potentially get treated.

Complications that can result from Shingles

The fact that Shingles results in an itchy rash often leads to infection, people can't seem to resist scratching and spreading the virus (and working against the body in the process by the way). For that reason, the following infections may result in approximately 1 in 20 cases of Shingle sufferers:

Bacterial Skin Infection

Many of us have had this before, and it's what our mothers all warned us about. "Don't scratch that – it'll get infected!" By scratching the rash, you actually only really serve yourself with temporary relief – and a handful of bacteria. By continually scratching, you will only reserve this bacteria to your body, which often leads to infections on the surface of the skin. A condition by the way, that will only prolong the itchy rash.

Hutchinson's Sign

When you see a blister on your nose, or note your eye is swollen, you have Hutchinson's Sign. This condition causes swelling, and can lead to total blindness if untreated.

Infected Organs

This has less to do with scratching and more to do with your internal health. When your immune system is failing, the virus gets to spread (rules of war). This can lead to extremely serious infections of very important organs, and because it likely indicates an already weakened immune system...can be fatal. If your Shingles hasn't already been treated, it's critical that you work to treat it – and to keep treating it so that it cannot spread. Seek medical attention if you haven't already to assess whether this may be the case.

Postherpetic Neuralgia (PHN)
This condition prolongs the length of Shingles disease because of the way it affects your cells. It desensitizes them and damages your nerves, making the brain less likely to provide the body with the resources it needs to fight off Shingles.

Unfortunately, this is also extremely common in those who suffer from Shingles and causes an extreme amount of pain in inactive as well as in active periods of Shingles.

Ramsay Hunt Syndrome
This is often identified as a form of ear pain, and occurs when the rash spreads to the face and ear. The ultimate consequences can be hearing loss, facial paralysis, and increased dizziness – so seek help if the virus spreads upwards!

The moral of the story? Do not scratch your rashes! Additionally, if you are in an active period of Shingles, wash your hands frequently and keep shorter fingernails – so that if you do wind up inadvertently scratching, the virus has fewer places to hide and thus less chance to spread.

In terms of how to know when infection has started to get serious, please consider the following list of symptoms, the presence of any of which should indicate the need to seek immediate medical attention:

- Dizziness
- Increased stiffness in the neck
- Infected rash
- Possessing a fever of 102 degrees Fahrenheit plus
- Possessing an extended fever, one that lasts longer than a week

- Rash on the eyes
- Tremors
- Vomiting or coughing more than before

Why the Rash?

So you may be wondering what exactly about Shingles causes a rash, well, the truth is, your body does. When the body senses the presence of any intruding cell that it did not create, it attacks it. This is a defence mechanism to help you battle infection, and is largely a good thing. It can cause physical effects however, like weakening of the immune system (because it's tired from fighting), fatigue in the body, and sometimes fever.

The rashes that are present with Shingles are actually little blistery sacks filled with fluid by the body (unpleasant to think of I know, but stay with me). The reason they fill with fluid is to alert the brain of the fight that's going on, to get more bodily resources involved.

The good news here is that the worse you feel, the harder your body is fighting the disease.

A Word on the Shingle's Vaccination

What are Vaccinations and how do they Help?
Vaccinations are where the body is injected with a weakened version of the disease it's trying to prevent so that the body can fight off the disease and become better at it, without ever having to suffer.

Where do you get Injections?
Injections are usually provided into the upper arm, and Zostavax is no exception. The difference here is that while we usually associate vaccinations with infancy, Zostavax is given only to those 60 years of age and older (as they are increasingly vulnerable to the effects of Shingles).

The Research Behind It
Clinical trials of 38,000 American seniors, half receiving Zostavax, half receiving placebo revealed that vaccination reduces Shingle's risk in seniors by 50%. Additionally, those who did get Shingles after the vaccination also had significantly shorter of a duration of pain that often comes with Shingles. This is quite impressive when you consider the fact that these participants were followed for three years on average, and studied for severity of Shingles and presence of Shingles.

Interestingly, the vaccination is less effective as individuals keep aging beyond 60, with efficacy reaching its peak at 64% if vaccinated between 60-69, and declining to 18% if given when the individual is 80+.

The Shingle's vaccination, Zostavax, has been widely open to the public since May 25, 2006.

Who Should be Vaccinated?

As YouTube documentaries will tell you, there are extremely conflicting ideas as to whether or not "every one" should be vaccinated. On the one hand, there are natural things you can do to prevent Shingles (see some of the tips in our guide for example) and there is some risk in infecting people to hope they can fight it off, but on the other hand the research has supported Zostavax as being extremely effective.

It's a personal decision as to whether or not you should be vaccinated, and one thing we can guarantee is that you should do research first to understand what is in the vaccination and the potential side effects.

Who Should not be Vaccinated

No vaccination works for every person, and Zostavax is no exception. The following is a list of vulnerable people groups who should not be vaccinated:

- Allergy sufferers – specifically those who suffer from an allergy to neomycin, gelatin, or the other components of Zostavax.

- Individuals whose immune system is already weakened by disease, medication, or blood disorders.

- Pregnant women

- Tuberculosis sufferers (when active).

The Importance of Understanding

Understanding Shingles is a huge part of enabling you to treat it, so we've taken the time to lay out the chapters above. Feel free to review whenever you're looking to learn more about what's going on, or when you're assessing if some one you love may be suffering. That being said, this is not a textbook, so we're done explaining what the disease is. It's time to move on to how to fix it!

Treating Shingles

We've learned a lot already about what Shingles is, but if you already know you have it, you're likely looking for the promised Shingles treatments. Don't worry, we're headed in that direction right now.

Let's take some time now and look into the treatment of Shingles – what we're all here for no doubt! This guide will focus on two elements of curing it, actually treating the disease, and ways to strengthen your immune system so it can fight it off. These elements go hand in hand.

Each chapter that follows this one is going to address methods of treatment, instructions for implementing those methods, and we'll finish up with an action plan for your personal case. As we go through the methods, keep a notepad handy in case you see something you need to add to your grocery list or find in your kitchen.

This guide will provide the knowledge you will need to treat Shingles, you've got the willpower to get your hands on the tools and actually be treated.

Sound good? Let's go then!

14 Popular Home Remedies for Shingles

This section is going to focus on home remedies. Home remedies have been recognized for centuries as being able to work to better individuals' health and well-being. Don't knock the power of the natural, sometimes the body just needs a little bit of help to trigger what it can already do itself.

These treatments are effective, and they're natural! You won't be putting harmful chemicals in your body to try to rid yourself of disease, and you won't be suffering any nasty side effects.

Another benefit of home remedies is that they often work with things you naturally have in your kitchen, or can cheaply obtain, making the treatment for Shingles accessible to all!

People are becoming increasingly willing to recognize the wisdom of home remedies, and that is why this guide has looked to them to help with this disease.

Aloe Vera Gel
Aloe Vera is a naturally occurring plant which has excellent anti-septic properties and medicinal qualities. It is often topically applied, and is a great anti-irritant for the skin, but also works internally in the form of stomach issues because of its anti-bacterial properties.

This may sound familiar to you, but aloe vera is an extremely valuable healing herb. It has been known to us since the days of the bible, and has many uses.

It has been used most commonly for skin irritations, infections, gastrointestinal distress, irritable bowel syndrome, and – most importantly to us – the curing of Shingles.

Find it at your grocery store, pharmacy, or health food store (I like Pure Aloe Vera Gel by Aubrey Organics).

Instructions

Step 1) Directly apply the gel onto areas of rash and infection. Aloe vera gel both acts as an anti-irritant and an anti-bacterial, so it will help you feel better and cure Shingles at the same time. Because of its gelatin nature, it also helps to ease the damage rashes can do to the skin, and prevents scarring.

Step 2) Continually apply 2-3 times per day until healed

Apple Cider Vinegar
Apple cider vinegar is created by fermenting the juices of an apple, and fermenting that by-product into apple cider vinegar. You can purchase the finished product from grocery stores or health food stores, depending on your area, to save you the work.

The many uses of apple cider vinegar
- Acne
- Arthritis aid
- Blood pressure balancer
- Chicken pox cure
- Hair care (prevents dandruff, provides shine)
- Mosquito bites
- Strengthening of the body
- Sunburns
- Toner for the face
- Those who suffer from acid reflux
- Throat aid

- Weight loss
- Yeast infections

"An apple a day keeps the doctor away"

We've all heard it. We've all repeated it! And indeed, apples do have some wonderfully naturally induced properties to help us. You see, apples contain acids and enzymes that are good for our general health, and can also help to cure Shingles.

Method 1: Drinking

Instructions

Step 1) Drink 1 tbsp. of apple cider vinegar every day, to promote a healthier you – which will help you fight off Shingles.

Step 2) Enjoy your newly cured body!

Method 2: Direct application

Instructions

Step 1) Using a sponge, gently dab the areas around the rash with apple cider vinegar.

Method 3: Bathing

Instructions

Step 1) Pour a bath

Step 2) Add 1/2 cup – 1 cup of apple cider vinegar

Step 3) Add tbsp. sea salt

Step 4) Stay in the bath for 20 minutes

Step 5) Gently towel dry

Baking Soda

Something that almost every kitchen already has, especially if there's a baker in the house, is baking soda. It is an extremely common ingredient throughout baking recipes and home remedies alike, and has been since its invention in the 1500s by Alfred Stock.

So what makes it so great? Well, besides its ability to raise a good cookie, it also has been known to have beauty properties, has been known to lower acidity within the body, and can balance PH levels.

There are multiple ways to use baking soda to cure shingles, and we are going to address both of them.

1) Baking soda blister help

2) Baking soda baths

Baking soda blister help

Step 1) Stir a few tbsp. of baking soda into lukewarm water.

Step 2) Using a sponge, gently apply the water to the areas of your body most effected by Shingle's

This paste has been known to quicken the healing of blisters and reduce the itchiness as it restores the PH levels to normal.

Baking soda baths

Step 1) Pour a remedy bath

Step 2) Add your oatmeal or malt vinegar (see below for instructions on preparing those for the baht).

Step 3) Add 1/2 cup of baking soda and mix into the water

Step 4) Remain 20 minutes

Step 5) Gently towel dry

Step 6) Lotion gently

Malt Vinegar Baths

So, as the name suggests this is a bath containing malt vinegar. Why malt? Because malt vinegar has been derived from barley, the process of its creation enables it to kill off many a virus. It's going to be recommended that you take one such bath every few hours while you're suffering until it stops it.

Instructions

Step 1) Pour yourself a nice warm relaxing bath

Step 2) Pour 1/2 cup of malt vinegar into the water, allowing it to mix thoroughly.

Step 3) Climb into the bathtub, paying particular attention that your rash gets coated in the water.

Step 4) Remain in the bathtub for 20 minutes at least. Read a good book, take some time to think, whatever you need to do to stay there.

Step 5) Drain the bathwater, rinse the tub, and gently towel dry. *It is critical here that you do not touch your rash, the blisters will be extremely sensitive.*

Step 6) Rub some lotion on the rash (I will recommend some just a bit later).

Frequency

Bathe in these baths at least every few hours until your rash lessens.

What else malt vinegar baths work for?

Malt vinegar is good for more than just treating Shingles. In fact, other things that malt vinegar is good for combatting includes: gout, kidney stones, sores, urinary tract infections, and of course – Shingles.

It's also easy and relatively cheap to obtain at any local grocery store, or even from Amazon.com (I like Organic Brown Rice Vinegar).

Oatmeal Baths

Oatmeal baths are another form of treating yourself just by taking a bath. If you'd like, you can alternate between malt vinegar and oatmeal baths to see which is the most effective for your Shingles, but you can use one or the other as well.

Oatmeal has the added bonus of likely already being in your cupboard, but on the off chance it's not, head out and pick up a bag. And it's cheap, so if you do have to pick it up, you needn't worry.

Instructions

Step 1) Take 1/3 cup of oatmeal and pour it into your blender.

Step 2) Set the blender to powder

Step 3) Test to ensure you have powdered sufficiently by stirring 1 tbsp. into warm water to check for absorption. Absorption = powdered just right, but if the water just sits there, you have a bit more to do.

Step 4) Pour a bath of lukewarm water.

Step 5) Pour the oatmeal into the bath, trying to distribute as evenly as possible.

Step 6) Wait a few minutes for the oatmeal to soak up the water. The bath should look milky before you climb in.

Step 7) Like with the malt vinegar bath, you need to climb in for at least 20 minutes.

Step 8) Drain the bathtub and rinse yourself completely off with warm water (oatmeal can be itchy if not washed out).

Step 9) Towel dry gently, again avoiding your sores as much as possible.

Step 10) Lotion.

Frequency
Every few hours, the same as the vinegar bath.

Chamomile
Chamomile has a very important active ingredient, bisabolol. Because of this active ingredient, chamomile can lay claim to anti-inflammatory, anti-microbial, and anti-irritant properties alike.

It is most often used in treatments of:
- Anxiety disorders and panic attacks
- Burns
- Diaper rash
- Flu
- Insomnia
- Menstrual cramps
- Muscular twitch issues
- Scrapes
- Skin conditions
- Ulcers

Because of chamomile's many uses, it is also widely available. You can find chamomile tea or chamomile lotions at your grocery store, your pharmacy, your health centre, or again online!

Chamomile baths
Step 1) In a small bowl, mix 2 tbsp. of dried chamomile flower and 1/4 cup of baking soda

Step 2) Mix in 1/2 tbsp. of honey

Step 3) Add 2-6 tbsp. of almond oil, little bit by little bit, until completely stirred in. This will make a little bath ball that you can simply drop into your warm bath for it to take effect!

Chamomile tea

Step 1) Place a purchased chamomile tea teabag in the bottom of a cup.

Step 2) Boil water for tea

Step 3) Steep the tea

Step 4) Drink

Chamomile tea is inherently relaxing, especially when you're drinking decaffeinated, and is often recommend in two cup dosages about one hour before you try to sleep.

Green Pea Water

Green peas are cheap, they taste great, and apparently they can also help with your Shingles. Let's take a look at how

Instructions

Step 1) Boil green peas on the stove, continuing until they're soft/cooked.

Step 2) Place a glass and drain the water from the pot into the glass

Step 3) Give the water time to cool, as it has just been boiling. THIS IS IMPORTANT, you can burn yourself if you rush this process.

Step 4) Using a sponge, gently dab the infected areas with the water – or take another bath and add this.

Honey

Honey, in its organic and natural form, is one of the best home treatments for many ailments – including Shingles! It is both anti-bacterial and anti-fungal, so it's great for many health issues.

Benefits of honey

- Acts as an aid to arthritis sufferers
- Allergy aid
- Battles bacteria
- Helps fight insomnia
- Combats colds
- Increases calcium absorption
- Promotes healthy hemoglobin count
- Promotes gastrointestinal health
- Relieves constipation

You can get it at your grocery store, you can get it at your healthy eating store, you can get it on Amazon (see Super Raw Honey by Wee Bee). The point is, it's easy to obtain and it works.

Let's see how.

Step 1) Take the honey and apply it to your infected areas on the skin.

Step 2) Allow the honey to seep into your skin. This usually takes between half an hour and an hour.

Step 3) Rinse the skin if it hasn't all seeped in.

Step 4) Gently towel dab (not rub) over the affected area.

Lemon Balm Tea

This herb has been a favourite for thousands of years. From its uses in France, to with the English and beyond, it is frequently called in to deal with issues related to headaches, depression, nerve pain, anxiety and yes, Shingles.

The herbs potency comes from its antioxidant properties, among other things, which essentially equip the body to battle off these issues. The wonderful thing is that because it is equipping the body to fight, it is still curing you – even as it makes you feel better. So you get the best of both worlds that way.

Lemon balm tea is probably going to become one of your favourite remedies because of its ability to battle off nerve pain, reducing the pain associated with your rashes as it cures them. It can be applied in conjunction with another antioxidant rich herb set (zinc and selenium any one?), but it can also be applied on its own.

Instructions:

Step 1) Boil some water

Step 2) Place 1 tbsp. of dried lemon balm leaves into the boiling water – as it boils – for around 15 minutes

Step 3) Remove from heat, and give time to cool!

Step 4) Using a sponge, gently (only use dabbing, you don't want to pop the blisters) apply this balm on the infections between three and four times per day.

Mint Leaves and Acetone (nail polish remover)

Mint was first located in India, the Middle East, and Europe, and has since become popular worldwide as a cure for Shingles and other disorders.

Mint has a lot of benefits people don't always get the chance to hear about. On top of smelling that fun minty fresh smell, it also has curative properties for many a health issue, and it doesn't taste that bad to boot.

That being said, the solution we will be mixing will be mixed with acetone (found in nail polish remover), so you **will not be drinking it.** Drinking acetone can cause significant harm. The reason we are adding the acetone is to add to the cure's strength and potency.

Instructions

Step 1) Convert four mint leaves to paste

Step 2) Mix in a cap full of nail polish remover

Step 3) Sponge over the rash you're suffering from

Step 4) Leave it alone. It will dry, and you can rinse if necessary then.

Neem Leaves

Everyone I have ever known who has known about Neem Leaves sings their praises. Neem leaves are a great treatment for Shingles, and they are one of the few treatments that can be used in many ways. You can make Neem Leaf tea, use it in a bath, take it as a supplement, or even find it in some creams. The unfortunate difference is you have to look a bit harder to find it, but if you want to skip heading to the Indian and Asian health food stores you can always buy dried Neem leaves or Neem Leaf oil cream fairly cheaply on Amazon.

> *NOTE: Pregnant women should not be using Neem Leaves. There has not been enough research done on the side effects to say it is safe.*

Neem leaves are used in the treatment of several skin conditions, boils, and even acne. Neem leaves also are involved in purifying blood and promoting better circulation, as well as the health of the immune system itself (one of the reasons it's so great with curing

Shingles), respiratory systems, and even malaria. Shingles victims have often been cured in just a few days with Neem Leaf!

The truth is that there's hardly room to discuss all of the areas of the body that Neem leaves are good for. If you're interested in hearing even more, look into Neem: The Ultimate Herb (by John Conrick) or Neem: India's Miraculous Healing Plant. These are both excellent reading material that will give you an even better understanding of this miracle herb.

For now, we will proceed with letting you know the ways you can use Neem Leaves to cure Shingles!

Method 1: Neem Leaf bath

    Step 1) Boil 100grams of Neem Leaves

    Step 2) Pour a bath, lukewarm is fine

    Step 3) Add the boiling water

    Step 4) Allow to cool to an acceptable temperature, then get in and wait your 20 minutes out (relax, enjoy, wash, etc.).

    Step 5) Gently towel dry

As with our other cures, you can add this to your oatmeal bath or malt vinegar bath.

Method 2: Eating Neem Leaf

You can simply indulge by eating Neem Leaf if you'd like, although if you'd rather consider one of the other methods it will be just as effective.

Method 3: Neem Leaf tea

    Step 1) Place 1 tsp. of Neem Leaf into a cup

    Step 2) Boil water

Step 3) Use the boiling water to make tea, allowing it to brew for a few moments before drinking.

Oil of Oregano

The oil of oregano plant comes in three different varieties: origanum acutidens, origanum minutiflorum, and origanum vulgare.

These plants have all been found in Turkey. Oil of oregano originated in the Mediterranean, but has since been exported all over the world for its natural antibiotic medicinal properties.

Benefits of Oil of Oregano

- To the stomach and gastrointestinal system
- To the immune system
- To the muscles
- To the skin

Research done in 2004 demonstrated the newly discovered fact that oil of oregano has antibacterial properties, and is capable of fighting some of the most concerning stomach bacteria, and also that it has been used to help herpes because of its similar antiviral properties. To date, we now know that it has antibacterial, antiviral, and anti-fungal applications.

It is used in treating infections, issues with bugs, and reducing the number of free radical cells. It is also used to strengthen the immune system and to help fight off infection, which is why it's so helpful in the curing of Shingles.

In terms of where you can find it, check your local pharmacy or health food store, or buy online (I like Global Healing Centre's website for their Oregano oil).

Instructions for applying oil of oregano will vary from brand to brand, so focus on the bottle of your particular brand for detailed instructions.

Step 1) Take X drops, X times per day orally.

Sandalwood Oil

Sandalwood oil works primarily because of its ability to help cool the body, which makes it harder for bacteria to thrive. It has many health related applications, but of course, we are most concerned with how it's going to cure Shingles!

Sandalwood oil should be applied three times per day until the rashes are gone. This is another oil that I recommend using after the bath (picking vitamin e oil, or sandalwood, would help your rashes heal faster).

In terms of where you will find it, you'll probably need to either purchase on Amazon or head to your local health food store – as it is not typically carried in pharmacies or grocery stores.

Instructions:

Step 1 (the only step)) Rub lightly and gently into the infected skin, giving it time to absorb in (do not rinse).

Use it again a few times per day, particularly when your wounds throb/feel warmer.

Vitamin E Oil

Vitamin E oil is a topically applied cure for Shingles. This is for a few reasons: it acts as an anti-inflammatory, it is rich in antioxidants, it has healing capabilities, and it can protect the skin from damaging itself during a rash.

NOTE: Vitamin E oil works great as a lotion, and can be used in the after bath application we have referenced in so many of our bathing instructions. In fact, I recommend it!

Vitamin E oil is also fantastic for reducing existing scars, as is aloe vera which we have already mentioned!

Instructions

Step 1) Take a bath, using the bathing instructions for your chosen method from above.

Step 2) Apply vitamin E oil.

About Bathing to Cure Shingles...

So you may have noticed we listed several baths in the chapter above. Let's take a minute and see how many you remember. Close your eyes and try to count how many before taking a peek at this list:

Ready? Check how many you got.

Types of Shingle curing baths
- Apple cider vinegar bath
- Baking soda bath
- Chamomile bath
- Green pea water
- Malt vinegar bath
- Neem Leaves bath
- Oatmeal bath

Whether you remembered or you didn't, the point is that each of these baths has curative properties – for Shingles and for other health issues.

Where you can get the ingredients:

I mostly stuck to baths that had staple ingredients many of your kitchens already have, but if they don't, head on down to the grocery store – or even purchase things online – to find all of the herbs and ingredients you need to be well on your way to a cure.

Reminder of frequency:

Though it is mentioned repeatedly above, I will remind you that these baths should be indulged in every few hours, for at least 20 minutes a time, until your rashes disappear. This will enable the herbs and ingredients to really get to the heart of the problem, and help you to feel better and get better, faster.

Benefits of bathing:

The added bonus to taking a bath to cure Shingles is once again that it is completely natural, there is nothing that's going to harm you about a little oatmeal water. (Just don't get in when boiling water has JUST been added, ha-ha, make sure the bath stays at an adequately warm but not hot temperature for you).

This can be a time for you to relax and enjoy yourself as well as to cure your Shingles. Bet you didn't think you'd hear that sentence, huh?

In terms of which bath is most effective, it varies from individual to individual. You may want to mix a few, you may want to just try individual ones until you figure out what works best.

I recommend starting to see which base works best and adding after that point, to increase your efficacy.

The bottom line is this: you can be cured of Shingles, and baths are a huge part of that process.

Supplements that have been known to Cure Shingles

Now that we've talked a lot about the natural herbs and baths you can take to cure Shingles, I'd like to take a moment and address some of the most popular supplements you can take to help.

Your body will be consuming energy and nutrients at a greater rate than usual when you're suffering from disease. This makes sense, and is why you will need to work hard (through diet and cures above) to get extra resources to your body. These resources enable your body to continue to fight, and to fight stronger against the Shingles virus.

Supplements are defined as "something added to a complete thing, to make up for a deficiency or to extend the strength of the whole".

Supplements, as the name suggests, can be a great way to add on to your plan to cure Shingles. Many of these can be found at your local health foods store or online, and I will be sure to pick accessible examples.

If you've found another supplement you'd like to try that is okay, just make sure that the phrase "buyer beware" definitely applies here. It is absolutely critical that you read the label when you're purchasing a supplement.

The reason to read the label? To know if it can help, and in what way. There are too many chalky pills being sold as cheap 'supplements' that really do nothing but make you feel like you've helped yourself. Don't be taken in. Research a high quality supplement, and don't be afraid to go for a higher price point – your body is not something you want to be cheap with.

This guide will highlight three supplements that have been shown to have a significant effect on Shingles. Please note that you can get these vitamins in your daily diet without supplements, supplements are just something to add on if you don't feel like you are getting enough of something in your diet.

Minerals
Minerals can be obtained through your diet, however if you know that you are lacking in one or more mineral supplements can be a great way to make up for the loss.

Minerals are critical to the body because of what they do for our metabolism. Our metabolism regulates converting broken down food into energy for the body and newer, healthier cells. When we are deficient in one or another mineral, there will be a huge impact on the body – especially when you consider the research on how closely various minerals work together and rely on each other.

Being deficient in one mineral could lead to other deficiencies easily!

Minerals are also extremely rich in antioxidants. We've talked a lot about the fact that you want this in an herb or food, but let's take a minute here and address why.

Antioxidants help in the breaking down of what's called "free radical cells". Free radical cells are actually cells packed with chemicals that can act like mini time bombs, prepared to release dangerous chemicals or wreak general havoc within the body at any time. Antioxidants prevent the formation of new free radical cells, and generally are able to fight existing ones.

This means that minerals are vital to keeping your body battling Shingles. If you think that you may not be getting enough minerals in your daily diet, don't be afraid to take a supplement to keep yourself on track.

I recommend Morningstar Minerals Energy Boost.

Multivitamin Supplements
As the name suggests, multivitamins contain combinations of the different vitamin groups. Your body needs a variety of vitamins (A, B12, C, D, E, K, and 7B complex vitamins) to regulate itself efficiently. When a person suffers from a lack in one of the vitamin groups, we call this a deficiency.

Vitamin deficiencies have serious health effects, but most important to us, your body does not function as well as it can – nor does your immune system – when it has a deficiency. This means that you will not be fighting off infections or diseases as easily as you could be, and the Shingles virus will be given free roam in your body if you do not correct it with dietary changes or a supplement.

Many people elect to take multivitamins, differing depending on the needs they want to fulfil. It's an easy and efficient way to get the nutrients your body needs, without necessarily having to eat five times per day. Multivitamins also each have different health benefits, from skin protection to heart health increase, to even just providing the body with more antioxidants or iron.

If you are considering taking a multivitamin, do your research beforehand to determine what grouping you will be looking for, and then head online or to the local health food store to pick up your supplement today!

Vitamin C Supplements
Vitamin C is something we've already talked about as being critical to the fight against Shingles.

What makes it so great?

- Antioxidant rich vitamin
- Dental hygiene (healthy gums)
- Strengthens the immune system
- Prevents future infections (and colds)

Vitamin C works to help your body heal faster primarily by strengthening the immune system, and providing antioxidants.

The reason vitamin C is taken sometimes as a supplement is because our body does not naturally produce it, and we lose it easily with the urination process.

You can get your Vitamin C intake from your diet, through many foods we will talk about in just a bit here, or through supplements.

If you have elected to use Vitamin C supplements, head out to your local health food store or online to Amazon and pick up a supplement today. Just be aware of the guidelines on individual dosages, as too much of any good thing isn't good for you.

Conclusions about Supplements

Supplements are for just what they're named, to supplement an existing system. You can get every vitamin and mineral that your body needs to fight Shingles via a healthy diet, but if you do notice you're still lacking in one or more vitamins or minerals, supplements can be a great way to get you on track.

Consult a family physician if you think that you are experiencing symptoms as the result of a vitamin or mineral deficiency, as they will be able to tell you concretely how much more of that substance you will need in a supplement.

We will be discussing how to create a healthier diet later, but in terms of supplements, head out to your local health centre or online to Amazon to find your supplements today.

Dietary Solutions for Shingles

Didn't know you could use food to help your body fight off Shingles? Well now you do! This chapter is going to overview a lot of simple to make foods that can help enable your body to cure you.

Don't forget, your body is already trying to rid itself of Shingles – it may just need a little help. Some of the best help you can provide comes in the form of nutrients and minerals that support your immune system, and that's what we're going to talk about here.

The added bonus? Eating healthier has benefits far beyond curing Shingles. You'll be feeling better eating cleaner, healthier foods – and getting better at the same time.

I recommend working the foods from this chapter into your diet for at least as long as you are suffering from Shingles, but you may well find you want to continue with them afterwards just for how they make you feel. This is great news! The healthier you are, the better your body is equipped, now and in the future.

Ever heard the phrase "we are what we eat"? Well, let's try eating some strength to fight off infection, some energy enhancing foods. What we're looking into here is providing the body with the supplies it needs, much in the way an army is supplied by its government.

So let's jump right in, here's our first food:

Cranberry Juice
What's so great about it?

- Organic cranberry juice is totally natural

- Liquids help to recover from Shingles. Even drinking more water will help you to heal faster than if you dehydrate.

How often should I drink it?

You should be drinking a 10-12 oz. glass of organic cranberry juice (mixed with the juices of a half a lemon for best effects) three times per day. This scheduling may fall best by drinking with each meal.

Where can I find it? Hit up the health food store for the best organic cranberry juice. You want to be sure you're avoiding preservatives and pesticides, as there's no telling what that will do to the efficacy of the cure.

Herbal Tea – particularly with added lemon or honey (or both)
What's so great about it?

- Herbal tea has been linked to many health benefits on top of its ability to help the body cure Shingles, not the least of which being polyphenols. Polyphenols are an antioxidant that has been linked to the reduction of risk of cancer.

- Herbal tea acts as an anti-inflammatory, which once again works to reduce swelling and improve the general functioning levels of the body.

- Tea is a liquid, again helping you to stay hydrated. We've talked about this all throughout the book, and we're not going to stop now.

Where can I find it?

You can find herbal tea at your local grocery store or health food store. To determine the quality of the tea, look for less caffeine and the presence of nutrients.

Add lemon or honey from your local grocery store for both flavour and added benefits (see their sections in this guide too for more information on the added benefits you can get from them).

How often should I be drinking it? This is another great once a day food. Make it a part of your after dinner routine, have a cup of herbal tea and relax.

Kiwi

What's great about kiwi?

- Kiwis are a source of several vitamins and nutrients that work to equip your body.

- On top of those, kiwis also provide digestive enzymes that help your body to process food. This will increase the effectiveness of ingesting other foods, as you will be digesting them properly so the nutrients get there faster.

- Contemporary research (done in Italy) found that kiwis (when ingested 5-7 times per week) reduced a child's likelihood of having difficulties wheezing, shortness of breath, or chronic bouts of coughing. This seems to indicate that kiwis have something to do with the health of your respiratory tract, something that can be attributed to the vitamin C and other substances we still don't fully understand in the kiwi.

How often should you indulge?

Kiwis are delicious and help you cure your Shingles, how often do you think you should eat it? Ha-ha, but seriously, likely a few times per day.

Where can you find it?

Like a lot of the food in this chapter, you can find kiwis in your grocery store (in the fruit section).

Lemon Water

What's so great about it?

- Lemon is a great food that helps to cleanse the body of infections, whether in your throat or throughout the body. By mixing water and lemons together, you get the benefits of both.

  There's a lot I could say about lemons, but I think you're getting the point. If you do decide you want more information, feel free to head to your local library or just use the internet to find out more about the healing properties of lemons.

- It helps on the goal of staying hydrated – which is absolutely vital to any time you're suffering from illness or disease.

  Drinking fluids helps the body to purify itself through "flushing". This is why you are constantly told if you have a cold or infection of any kind to drink lots of fluids. Lemon water is delicious, and on top of the water going a long way to staying hydrated, the lemons also have the added benefits listed above – so you're getting the best of both worlds with very little effort.

  A note though: Make sure the water you're using is purified. You want to do this to get clean water, not water bogged down by chemicals and chlorine that you may just get from the tap. Bottled water is an acceptable solution to this, just don't forget the lemon! The lemon has all kinds of healing properties, and is the key to curing Shingles.

Where can I find it?

This should seem fairly obvious, but bottled water and lemons are both available at your local grocery store and often farmers market, which can be a great way to get fresh foods.

How much should I be drinking?

You should be drinking between 8-10 glasses of water every day, even without Shingles. When you have Shingles, the experts typically suggest about half an ounce per pound of body weight (so if you weigh 200 pounds you should be drinking 100 ounces).

This will be enough to keep you hydrated and have your body functioning well again in no time.

A word on water:

We cannot say it enough. Water is the key to curing disease and infection because it is a fluid. It will keep you urinating regularly, which is your body's chance to flush infection out, and it also replenishes your body's energy stores.

Did you know that your body is 70% weighed in with water? That's right, water is the key to life here. From flushing out the system, to carrying nutrients, to helping your body produce mucus and other infection battling elements, water is really what's going to help here.

We just wanted to take some time and emphasize the importance of this life saving liquid.

Smoothies

What's so great about smoothies?

In truth, like the vegetable juice we'll talk about later, the best thing about smoothies is that you get the benefits of multiple healthy foods all at once. They are also a delicious treat to brighten your day.

The main thing you will need for smoothies is the ingredients (we'll review some great ones in just a second), and a blender to smoothie the ingredients.

Each person has their own individual preferences as to what should go in a smoothie. While this guide will emphasize the importance of making it healthy foods only, we will make a wide list so that you can see the full range of choice that making smoothies really provides.

Healthy ingredients list for smoothies:
- Almond milk
- Fruit: Avocado, bananas, blueberries, blackberries, kiwis, raspberries, strawberries, watermelon, oranges, etc.
- Superfoods: Hemp, maca root, spirulina, and more.
- Vegetables: Broccoli, carrots, cucumber, lettuce, spinach, tomato

You can really put whatever you want into a smoothie, just make sure you're thinking about what that is and what health benefit it will have for you.

Where can I find them?
Smoothies can be made right in your own home, or at a juice bar or coffee shop. They have become increasingly popular because of their health benefits, so if they're something you enjoy rest assured that they're easy to get your hands on.

Soup
What makes it so great?
Soup is a very light weight meal. It will not bog your body down by taking up all its energy on digestion, but will still provide an adequate amount of nutrients – depending on the type of soup you make.

This guide will provide a recipe for Carrots and Coriander soup, because this combination has been found so extremely effect at getting rid of Shingle's rash.

Carrots and Coriander Soup

Ingredients

- 100 grams of carrots
- 60 grams of Coriander

Instructions

Step 1) Boil some water

Step 2) Add in 100 grams of carrot

Step 3) Time for the coriander. Stir in the 60 grams of Coriander

Step 4) Continue stirring and boiling for 30 minutes

Step 5) Strain the mixture into an awaiting glass or bowl, and drink up for your cure to Shingles!

Spinach

What's great about spinach?

- Spinach acts as an anti-inflammatory, which will help reduce swelling associated with rashes and internally ease your body's struggle.

- Spinach is a source of countless vitamins and minerals, including Vitamins A and C, folate, magnesium, and iron. Just by eating this one food, you empower your body already by strengthening it in a variety of ways – not the least of which is by strengthening your immune system.

- Spinach is rich in an antioxidant like substance called flavonoids. Contemporary science has told us that it has as many as thirteen different varieties of these substances, that will each work to help your body battle disease!

Where can you find it?

You can find it at your grocery store or local food store, and it often works in an nice salad.

So do what your mother always told you and eat your vegetables! Spinach helps a lot with the battle to cure Shingles through the nutrients, flavonoids, and vitamins that it contains.

Vegetable Juice
Vegetables, in their many forms, are one of the best things you can ingest to help your body fight off Shingles – and to be healthier. Whether you prefer broccoli, tomatoes, cucumber or carrots... you will be helping yourself.

The benefit of vegetable juice is it combines the powers of a lot of these veggies into one powerful drink. If you head to your local grocery store, you'll be sure to find several varieties of vegetable juice that can help you cure your Shingles, and feel better about yourself.

An alternative to buying premade juice is making your own. You will need a juicer and some vegetables, but it can be worth it to taste the freshness of something made by yourself right in front of you.

Another great way to get your daily dosage of vegetables is through a salad. Mix in what you'd like, add a little lemon or olive oil for flavouring, and voila. You've got a loaded serving of tomatoes, carrots, cucumbers, lettuce, lemon, and whatever else you chose to put in there.

Each of these vegetables has its own set of benefits and helps to curing Shingles, but the bottom line is that they strengthen your immune system – which enables it to fight all the harder. Make sure you're getting several servings of vegetables every day, whether in salad, smoothie, or juice form.

Wheatgrass
What's great about it?

- Wheatgrass is antibacterial in nature

- Wheatgrass has been known to produce balance within the

white cell and red cell count in your bloodstream, and thus to improve circulatory health.

- Wheatgrass helps to purify the body of toxins. In fact, Dr. Earp-Thomas (who works with Ann Wigmore) has gone on the record as having said that 15lbs of wheatgrass is the nutritional equivalent of 350 pounds of other vegetables in this regard.

- Wheatgrass is a highly oxygenated substance, promoting better tissue function.

- Wheatgrass is high in enzymes, particularly in juice form

- Wheatgrass promotes better liver functioning

- Wheatgrass and wheatgrass juice are great for the skin (when drank) because of their cleansing nature.

  In fact, you can pour the juice over your body and soak in a bath for 15-20 minutes, and you'll notice a difference in your skin.

- Wheatgrass provides the body with the light producing chlorophyll, the sustainer of plant life and helper of human life.

- Wheatgrass is a cure for sore throats

Where can I find it?

You can often find wheatgrass at juice bars, and remember you probably only need about one ounce per day to begin.

Wheatgrass may not be the best tasting substance, but it is one of the most potent cures for Shingles... and it has a lot of other health benefits we've discussed. I definitely recommend wheatgrass, and if it makes you feel any better about the taste? I drink it myself.

Yogurt

What's so great about it?

- Yogurt is easy to make, doesn't take anything to prepare, and is light on the stomach – so even if you don't feel like eating much you can likely get it down.

- Yogurt has been proven to be able to boost your body's immune system strength, naturally enabling you to fight off the Shingles.

- Yogurt is chalk full of nutrients: calcium, protein, riboflavin, and vitamins B12.

- Yogurt helps the digestive system, again increasing the effectiveness of ingesting other nutrient rich foods by making it easier for the body to digest.

- Probiotics are often referred to as the good bacteria, and with good reason. Probiotics go into the body and fight against bacteria (and all the infections that they cause as a result), this is the "bad bacteria" versus "good bacteria". Yogurt, as you may have heard, is absolutely packed with probiotics.

- Good source of liquid, 88% water

Where can you find it?

You can find yogurt at any grocery store and a lot of health food stores. Make sure to check the label for the most organic yogurt – it will be the one highest in probiotics – to avoid ending up with a sugary replica that doesn't help nearly as much.

How often should you be indulging? Once a day is a good place to start with yogurt.

Foods to Avoid when trying to Cure Shingles

We've been spending a lot of time discussing what you can do to get rid of your Shingles, but I want to stop now and take a quick bit of time to focus on what you need to avoid doing, eating poorly.

This chapter will list some of the worst food offenders. When you put junk into your body, it does not contain the nutrients to equip your immune system, it does not help, and worse – some junky foods can actually sap nutrients and energy. This takes energy away from your fight against Shingles, allowing the virus to thrive while your body is focused on breaking down whatever you decided to put in.

Neglecting to change your diet could be a big part of the reason why you're still struggling with Shingles today, so let's stop the process in its tracks.

Let's take a look at the foods you need to get off of your what to eat list!

Dairy Products
With the exception of yogurt, dairy products are all relatively unhelpful when battling Shingles. Though they don't qualify as "junk food", they do help the body to build up mucous. This can be good when trying to fight off say, a cold, but very bad when you need the nutrients not to be soaked up by your body's levels of mucous.

I recommend avoiding all dairy except yogurt throughout your struggle with Shingles. If you're looking for a replacement, try almond milk or rice milk.

Meat

Mean should be avoided because it weighs heavily on the digestive system's resources. As much as meat has its time and place, it's too hard on your system for the relatively low amount of nutrients it provides, and will only serve to suck up much needed resources in your body with the digestive process. You don't want to take away from your Shingles struggle, so focus on foods that are easier on the digestive tract and higher in nutrients to get the most out of your diet.

Sugar/ "junk food"

Junk food, as the name implies, is just that. These foods are high in sugar, fat, and cholesterol – and low in anything good for you. All that sugary foods does is hurt your body. In fact, junk foods are often acidic, which breaks down nutrients.

This is something you should always avoid wherever possible. Sugar binds your blood cells together, making blood flow more difficult and antibodies have to struggle more to get to the sites of the infections they're so heartily battling.

Avoid: junk food, ice cream, candy, and anything you know to be devoid of nutrients. We are beefing up your body's defence system – not interested in tearing it down!

A note about the sugar in fruits: Sugar in fruit is fine for the body, and has not been linked to damaging health benefits of any kind.

Medicinal Treatment of Shingles

I have gotten a lot of questions over the years about what medications work to treat Shingles. Personally, I have elected to opt for a more natural lifestyle, which is why most of this guide has been focused on completely natural and inexpensive cures, but I do recognize that there are those who would still seek medicinal intervention.

In fact, as we mentioned in our introduction, there are those for whom professional medical intervention is necessary (see the symptoms of Shingles chapter near the beginning of this guide). I do not object to this, and indeed I recommend you seek medicinal intervention if indeed you think you might need it.

One of the reasons we always recommend checking in with a medical professional before treating Shingles is for this very reason. We are not medical professionals, and this guide is not to substitute professional medical advice. Additionally, medical professionals can tell you for certain whether or not you require medicinal intervention or natural intervention. You can do both!

To that end, this chapter will review some of the medications that have had the most success in treating Shingles.

Acetaminophen
More commonly referred to as Tylenol, acetaminophen is a painkiller that works to alleviate the painful symptoms you may be having.

Please note that acetaminophen is not a cure for Shingles, but rather a medication to ease the pain you may be going through.

Acyclovir (Zovirax)
Acyclovir/Zovirax is a prescription strength anti-viral drug that will cure Shingles. Dosages usually require you to take the medication 5 times per day, and has seen some success.

It should be noted however, that most of the success of this drug comes if taken before the rash occurs. After the rash occurs, the antiviral still will get rid of your Shingles, but you may have to consult a natural remedy to deal with your rash.

Antihistamines
Over the counter antihistamines can be picked up at a pharmacy or you may require prescription strength.

They can help reduce the allergy like symptoms of Shingles, like swelling and pain.

Some of the best antihistamines are as follows:
- Atarax (hydroxyzine)
- Benadryl (diphenhydramine)

  *Both of the above have been known to incite tiredness and should only be taken in the evening.
- Allegra (fexofenadine)
- Claratin (loratadine)
- Zyrtec (certrizine)

While none of the three above listed have been known to cause drowsiness, they may require a prescription, so head out to the family doctor if you think these are what you need.

Calamine Lotion

This is an over the counter lotion that is often associated with chicken pox, poison oak, poison ivy, and more because of its ability to reduce itchiness and relieve rashes.

It acts as a soothing agent on the skin, and coats it as often as needed to prevent you from needing to scratch (and thus spreading the infection).

Famciclovir (Famvir) and Valacyclovir (Valtrex)

These are both antiviral drugs that can be prescribed to help the body fight off the infections associated with Shingles, like herpes, sores, chicken pox, and Shingles. It does not itself cure Shingles, but could give the body a better chance to clear out the infection itself by reducing the resources needed to combat complicating infections we've talked about as possible.

Conclusions about Medications and Products

Talk to your doctor if you've seen something about a medication or antihistamine that you think may be right for your symptoms. Over the counter items can always be tried, but it's often best to seek medical advice first.

Now that we have discovered natural cures for Shingles, and talked about medicinal cures for Shingles, we're going to take some time and discuss other types of products that have had some success with Shingles.

Other things to try with Shingles

You've probably already gotten this notion, but I have extensive experience with Shingles cures. I have done mountains of research, and I want you to be able to benefit from all of it.

I have already walked you through the natural cures for Shingles, the dietary aspects of Shingles, and medicinal options for Shingles treatment, but I want to take this chapter and discuss a few specific products I've run across that really seem to help alleviate it.

Aveeno Anti-Itch Concentrated Lotion with Natural Colloidal Oatmeal
I've recommended this in the past and had some great reviews. This guide has already gone over the power of oatmeal, and Aveeno's lotion puts that power to work in a nature based formula.

Force of Nature – Chicken Pox & Shingles Balm
Similarly, I heard about this product a while ago and got the chance to try it. As the name suggests, it has had success treating Shingles, so I feel comfortable recommending you head on over to Amazon and pick it up today if that's what you'd like to do.

Quick Relief: Easing the Pain of Shingles

The pain that comes with Shingles rashes can be intense. I often get asked, is there a way to relieve it instantly? I have a few suggestions to ease the pain of Shingles quickly, even before you start to work on a cure, and I thought I'd share them with you now.

One valid option is a painkilling medication, like acetaminophen or Advil. These pills may relieve the pain in as little as an hour, although they will not work to cure the underlying causes.

If you're like me though, you're always looking for the natural alternative. So here's a more natural way to ease your pain with low cost and effort:

Ice. You heard me. Just go down to the store and pick up an ice pack, and ice the rash you have for at least 20 minutes.

Ice numbs your body, so you won't be feeling any pain, and best of all? If you get two ice packs you can rotate them in the freezer so that one is out and one is being frozen, then the frozen is taken out and other cools again, so that you can have all day pain relief.

Another completely natural way for you to relax and ease the pain is just focusing on rest. Resting is the body's time to regenerate, and when you rest, your body gets to focus its attention where it's needed (in this case the pain). The one good thing about Shingles is it can remind you to slow down and take a break, read a book, or go researching on the internet.

Any of these options are valid ways to get rid of your pain, at least temporarily, but should not be thought of as cures. These are numbing and painkilling agents, to make the immediate sensation of pain go away, not the rash itself. Use them on the days things get bad – and don't be afraid to try aloe vera gel or the other cures mentioned at the same time!

Quick relief: How to Avoid Scratching the Rash that comes with Shingles

If you've ever had a Shingles rash, or you're experiencing one now, you will know just how itchy they get. As we have already talked about though, itching the rash only prolongs it – and even possibly spreads it depending on how often you wash your hands and how you keep your nails.

Scratching blisters risks popping them, which lessens the signals to the brain to send additional resources to that area – and thus lets the virus thrive even longer. Scratching also catches harmful bacteria up under your fingernails, and enables the virus to be passed anywhere you then touch.

Scratching can also lead to scarring and a lot of other complications – not the least of which is infection – but the bottom line is just to avoid it. We recognize this is easier said than done sometimes though, so we've written to help here.

This chapter will be dedicated to methods to avoid scratching that itch, so you can let your body get its work done without interruption.

Baths
We've talked already about several natural baths that can help alleviate your suffering and avoid scratching. Even taking a bath in just water should alleviate the instinct to itch somewhat, although you must be gentle when drying afterward or you will just end up irritating the rash all over again.

Using oven mitts

We've all seen it in cartoons, but in emergency situations sometimes this is the only way to stop yourself from scratching. Put on a pair of oven mitts and have some one tape them to your arms.

Taking Action: Formulating Your Plan for Curing Shingles

I know we've provided a lot of information in this guide. It wasn't intended to overwhelm, it was intended to give you options. However, I recognize that for some people, it can be tough to decide what to try first.

I know that there isn't enough time in the world to try everything, so I'm going to use this chapter to outline how you can make your own personalized action plan for how you will cure Shingles.

Step 1) Selecting the methods

You now know a lot of methods. Take out a sheet of paper, or open a word file, and write down the ones that have appealed to you most.

If you don't remember, head back to the previous chapters and just scan the headings, no need to re-read yet unless you're going to be using that method.

Some questions to ask yourself at this stage:

1) Do I want purely natural or also medicinal interventions?
2) How many of these ingredients/items do I already have in my home?
3) Where will I go to pick up these items? (Each chapter had a note on where to find the items required)

Step 2) Getting the ingredients/items

This is a simple but important step, because you can know oatmeal will help, but if you don't have any oatmeal... You get the picture.

Make a list before you go of the specific items you will need (based on the methods you've already selected) and the places you will need to go to get them. Don't forget you can get them online too if that's easier.

If you can't get out, ask a friend or family member to go out for you to grab the ingredients. If you'd rather keep your Shingles private, head to Amazon to order the things you'll need and you can have them delivered (often within the span of a day or two).

Step 3) Start with one of the baths

The baths are one of the fastest methods to naturally alleviate the itching and begin the process of ridding yourself of this terrible rash.

Set a few times per day that you can take these baths, and don't be afraid to mix and match the cures to see what works best for you!

It's also worth noting you will need to plan on towel dry and lotioning time after each bath, as that can add a few extra minutes you may not normally need.

Step 4) Select your lotion

If you haven't already, select a lotion to keep near the bathroom so that when you're finished and dry, you can apply it.

Make sure you have enough supply, a few bottles should be sufficient, to keep yourself from having to go out again and again while you're still suffering – as this can become frustrating.

Step 5) Dietary changes

Make a plan regarding your diet. Are you going to be changing anything? Do you have the required foods at home? Do you have foods you should be avoiding at home? Setting up your kitchen to support your fight against Shingles can be a big part of the action plan, so take your time and make notes here as needed.

Step 6) Hydrate, hydrate, HYDRATE!

We can't say it enough – liquid is what's going to save you here. It is through hydrating the body that you enable it to discard the wasted infectious cells, enabling new cells to take their place. Always be hydrating, whether with chamomile tea, herbal tea, water, lemon water, or even vegetable juice.

Calculate the exact amount of water you should be intaking, and make sure you get it!

Step 7) Anything else

This is the space where you should be planning for anything else. Book a doctor's appointment, write down your favourite methods to stop yourself from scratching, make plans to keep your needed cure items stocked in full supply.

The key to an action plan is, well, action. I've outlined the tools, but it's up to you to choose which ones you'll use and to make sure you're using them. I'm confident that as soon as you start to use these cures, you will see an impact – for most of you within just a few days.

So if you've followed along by now then it's time to be happy, it's time to cure your Shingles!

When will you know Your Shingles is gone?

As the rash is going to start disappearing, and the symptoms are going to start alleviating, you may be wondering – how will you know when it's finally over?

This chapter will review some of the signs and signals your body will give you to tell you it's time to party, your Shingles is gone.

Scabbing blisters
Scabbing blisters are a great sign, they indicate that the body has drained the moisture from the scabs (so you're probably feeling less itchy) and that the sores are preparing to fall off. The great news is, once all of the moisture is gone you will no longer be contagious either!

No more blisters
By the time your blisters are gone and your pain is removed, you will primarily be over the virus. It could still be in the process of being fought within the body, but it is on its final legs – it is defeated.

The key here is to keep to a consistent way of doing things until you're certain. My recommendation is to continue treatment until a few days after the last visible and physical signs of Shingles have left your body.

Once this is done, congratulate yourself – and get some rest. Rest will enable the body to recharge from the immense battle it's just been through. Be grateful that Mother Nature has provided us with so many different ways to naturally rid yourself of the disease, and celebrate!

Conclusions

If you've made it this far then you are well aware by now that you have in your head the power to cure Shingles. Congratulations!

I hope I've earned the trust that you placed in me by reading this book, and I hope you follow through and see that you can be free of your Shingles – that's what I really wanted to offer with this book, and that's what I hope you have received.

It's worth noting that this book can be used as a reference, any time you need a refresher on the methods or want to try a different one. I provided a lot of options so you could have a lot of options, so take the time to go back over chapters if you need to.

I wish you a speedy recovery, and a life of happiness!

Visit :
www.naturesnaturalhealth.com/join/
To Sign Up for our Exclusive Health Newsletter
TODAY!

Made in the USA
Lexington, KY
29 October 2015